Terms and Conditions

LEGAL NOTICE

The Publisher has strived to be as accurate and complete as possible in the creation of this report, notwithstanding the fact that he does not warrant or represent at any time that the contents within are accurate due to the rapidly changing nature of the Internet.

While all attempts have been made to verify information provided in this publication, the Publisher assumes no responsibility for errors, omissions, or contrary interpretation of the subject matter herein. Any perceived slights of specific persons, peoples, or organizations are unintentional.

In practical advice books, like anything else in life, there are no guarantees of income made. Readers are cautioned to reply on their own judgment about their individual circumstances to act accordingly.

This book is not intended for use as a source of legal, business, accounting or financial advice. All readers are advised to seek services of competent professionals in legal, business, accounting and finance fields.

You are encouraged to print this book for easy reading or read for free.

Table Of Contents

Foreword

Dance may have been created for enjoyment, aesthetic expression, and socialization; but these days, it is considered one of the most effective ways of exercising for fat loss. In this course – Dancing your Fats Away – you will learn some of the things that make dance or dancing an excellent method of getting fit and healthy. Get all the info you need here.

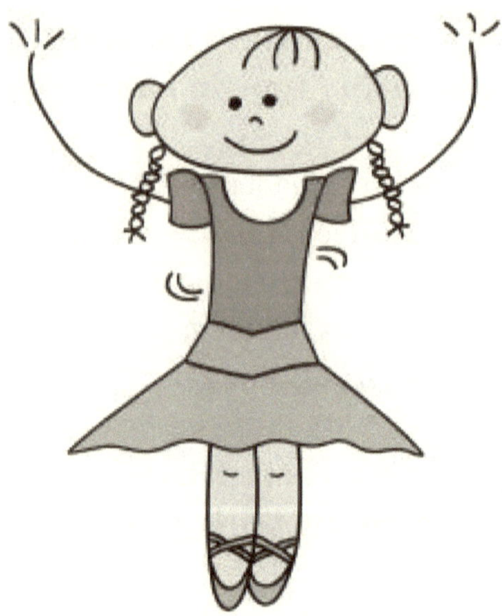

Dancing Your Fats Away
Things You Can Learn From Dancing Classes

Chapter 1:

Introduction

Synopsis

By reading through this course consisting of 10 short chapters, you will learn why dancing is a good workout for weight loss and what specific types of dances, dance moves and steps contribute to realization of that objective. You will read a case study (chapter 10) that sums up the lessons you can get from dancing as a method of losing weight.

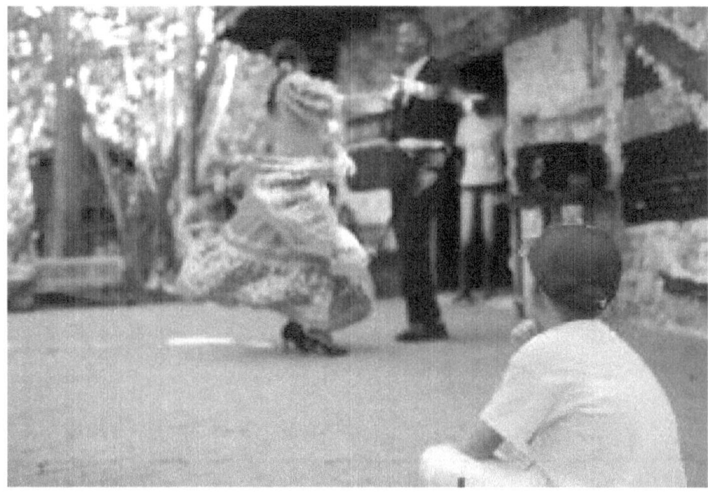

Course Preview

Gaining weight is easy; you eat a lot of calorie-rich foods, neglect exercises and that's it. The problem is that it is easy to get used to foods that induce weight gain and resting on the couch while watching your favorite program on TV. That is the reason why engaging in activities promoting fat loss requires a lot of willpower specially when the program you have chosen involves enduring low calorie diets and strenuous workouts. Of course, you probably do not know that there is an easier and more enjoyable way of working out; and that's dancing.

There are various kinds of dancing, some are slow and involves precise movements, and others are faster seemingly putting greater demands on the body. You would say that the faster dances are better for exercise, but it actually depends on the kinds of position a dance would require you to do. The more challenging the position, the more you get a proper workout.

Choosing The Right Dance

In case you are into a type that's fast, you can try hip-hop or salsa. If prefer slow dance, you can try ballet steps. Around 20 minutes every day of the dance of your choice should do wonders in getting you slimmer.

Select the type that will not put a lot of stress on your body especially if you are not getting any younger. And like any other workout, start with the easier moves and proceed to the more challenging ones only when your muscles have adapted to the physical activity.

Advantages Of Dancing For Fat Loss

The main advantage of dancing over other types of workouts is that it is not wearisome because you can actually like it. Anything that gives enjoyment is easier to do and more than this, you will probably be eager to do it.

Another advantage of dancing for burning fats is you can do it anywhere – inside your house, in a park nearby, or if you have a cubicle or a private office, in the workplace. People being social beings, it is even more enjoyable when you can do it with friends.

Besides the physical benefits that directly results from fat burning, dancing teaches you another important lesson – discipline. This helps you develop a deeper commitment to your fat loss diet and other things important to your life.

Chapter 2:

The Tricks Behind Dancing

Synopsis

Great dancers have a couple of tricks under their sleeves which help them become better dancers. Some may be very gifted or talented at dancing; but talent alone can only get you so far, some of the tricks, rather, tips discussed below are guaranteed to aid you in achieving satisfactory results.

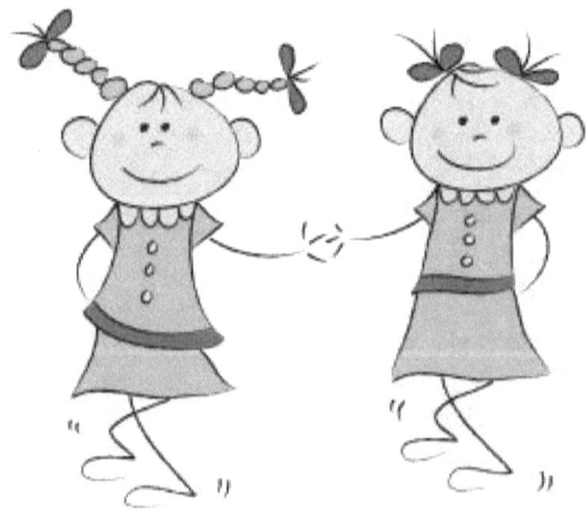

Find a Good Dance Coach

An experienced dancer knows all too well how valuable a good dance teacher is; an instructor not only teaches new dance moves or techniques but also helps to spot and correct mistakes. If you are one of those people who have been taking dancing lessons for some time but you never seem to improve, it may be time to find a new dance coach. You may embark on your search by checking the local dailies or the yellow pages for dance tutors; a number of universities offer evening dance classes at reasonable costs.

A good dance instructor should have been in the dancing business for a while and have some sort of dancing certification or qualifications. Ensure the teacher is qualified to teach the dance style of your choice; for instance, find out whether his/her forte lies in dance genres like jazz, hip-hop, modern, tap, or ballet.

Find an instructor who is proud of and dedicated to their craft, one who appears to be engrossed in the idea of teaching dance to their students. It goes without saying that your dance instructor should always be punctual for your sessions since a good dance teacher should strive to be a symbol of responsibility and excellence to their students.

Learn From Others

Watching other dancers, paying close attention to their techniques, posture and body alignment will help you grow as a dancer especially when you incorporate their moves into your dance routine. Dance movies can not only be entertaining but are also a great source of inspiration; some of them include Flashdance, Strictly Ballroom, Center Stage, Saturday Night Fever, Dirty Dancing, Mad Hot Ballroom, Save the Last Dance, Dance With Me, Shall We Dance, and Step Up.

Posture

Good posture involves standing up straight, pushing your shoulders back and down and then holding your head up high. Proper body alignment and posture is important as it helps dancers appear more confident if not elegant not to mention improving body control and overall balance. It is also one of the most vital aspects of dancing with a partner; slumping and slouching is not only bad for your health but it also reduces your level of alertness making you appear less confident.

Stretching

Stretching on a daily basis improves the flexibility of your body making your dance moves seem much more effortless since the more flexible your limbs, the easier it is for you to move them. Making a habit to do some stretches before dancing is an important step, though the most neglected, that will make a huge difference to your dancing. A good stretching routine should focus on your muscles, also bearing in mind that a light jog or easy walking is sufficient enough to warm up the leg muscles.

Relax

Most people do their best dancing when relaxed which can be achieved by taking in a couple of deep breaths and clearing your mind by unwinding to some good music. Start by sitting with your back straight and your feet on the floor; you should feel comfortable and alert. With your eyes closed, take in a deep breath through your nose and then exhale slowly, again through your nose. Repeat this process and remember to practice daily for about 20 minutes before your dance session, you can also have mini relaxations through-out the day, both at work or at home.

Shoes and Technique

Good technique separates a good dancer from the best dancer since a professional dancer dedicates a lot of their time trying to perfect their techniques; it is important to master new moves but also strive to perfect your skills in each step.

Each dance genre requires specific types of shoes; dance shoes have been carefully structured to offer protection to the feet and legs to the dancer's benefit. Ensure that you are using the right kind of shoes and that the shoes also fit well so as to avoid hurting yourself.

Chapter 3:

Why Dancing Is the Way to Go For Fat Loss

Synopsis

Any type of physical activity that a person does on a regular basis can result to weight loss. It can either be running, jogging, climbing up and down the stairs or using the exercise equipment on a gym. It will eventually help in losing the excess fat in a person's body.

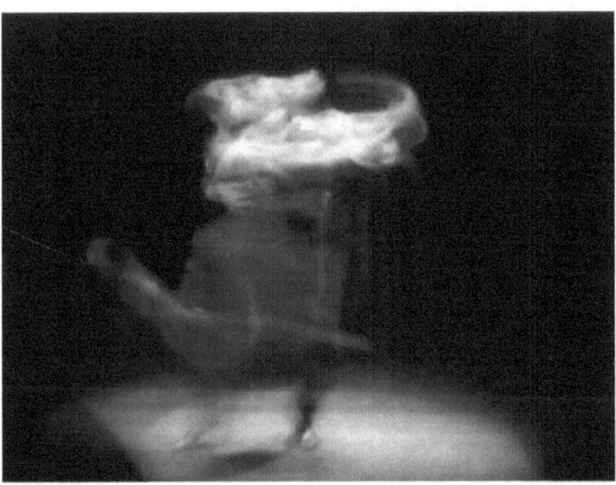

What Happens

If you are aiming to have a fitter body this 2013 but don't know what workout to do, why not consider dancing? Dancing is fun, creative and entertaining. Everyone can dance! Some lack the confidence, some lack rhythm, but everyone has the ability to learn.

Dancing is a type of aerobic exercise that can be done in a fast or slow pace, depending on what your body can handle. It is best done in a class with an instructor and other students so the risk of getting injured is low.

To be able to successfully lose weight by dancing, you should do it regularly. The right way to do it is to start with a warm up that can be done for at least five minutes. This will loosen up tight muscles in your body and help you move without hurting yourself. You should allow 30 minutes to an hour of dance at least 4 to 5 times a week. Depending on the intensity of your dance, you can lose up to 500 calories in just an hour session.

The best thing about dancing is that it's never boring. If one form of dance doesn't work for you, you can move on to a different one that fit your style and needs. There are different types of dances that you can try.

For instance, if you want something that is fast and can get your heart rate up in seconds, then zumba, hip hop or samba is the way to go.

For a slower, less intensity workout, there's ballet or jazz. If you want something more unique, try hoop dancing or pole dancing. All of these dances will lead to a slimmer, healthier version of yourself!

Dancing is pretty easy. Put on some music and move your body to the beat. The best part of it all is that if you are too embarrassed to let other people see you, you can still do it in the comforts of your own room. When done regularly, you can tone your muscles and have a stronger body. It is not just good for you physically but also emotionally. It is said that dancing can be a good form of stress reliever!

But like any other type of workout, it is best to do it with the right kind of diet. Surely, this is a great exercise but if you are constantly eating food that is not good for your body (high in cholesterol, low in vitamins), then you will have to work double time. Drinking a lot of water is also encouraged. Stay hydrated whenever you do any kind of physical activity.

If you are overweight or obese, it is best to consult a doctor before doing a heavy routine. They might have a workout routine that is better for you.

Chapter 4:
Dancing and Exercise Tips

Synopsis

Dancing is considered to be one of the most difficult athletic art forms, and it has a lot of distinction. Flexibility, skill, fitness, safety and satisfaction are the things that you will definitely obtain from your dancing experience, no matter what age you started dancing.

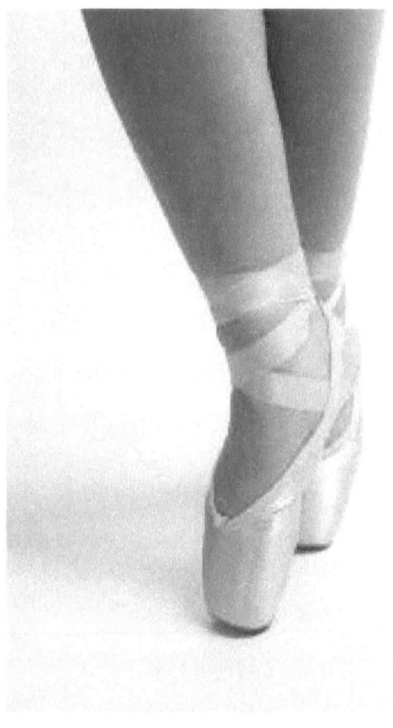

Tips

Shoes

Shoes play an important role in dancing. There is a wide variety of shoes that you can choose from. Let the dance instructors himself recommend the best shoes for you, for they know which ones are comfortable for your feet when you dance. Jumping, leaping, pirouetting, sliding and moving your feet to the beat have a big impact on your feet, ankles and shins. There are a lot of fashionable and stylish shoes available in stores today that can also help protect your feet.

Warming Up

Provide a little extra time to warm up before dancing. Make sure to arrive in dancing class a little earlier so you could do some warm ups first. Some stretching and exercising is needed before dancing to avoid any possible injuries. It is also recommended that you wear a sweatshirt while warming up so it can help the body stay warm.

Condition

Conditioning your body is also important. There are some programs that teach cardiovascular endurance, flexibility and versatility, and muscle strength training. If you are aiming to reduce weight by dancing, you should consult a doctor first. This is to make sure that you don't over exercise; and to help you maintain a pace that is suitable for your health condition.

Stretching

Do some stretching before and after sessions. Try to push your stretch enough to feel a pull, not pain. Try holding each stretch for 30 to 60 seconds. Muscle stretching will help improve and increase your flexibility.

Technique and Posture

According to the National Dance Association, having proper technique plays an important role in avoiding and eliminating possible injuries in dancing. Technique is the method that you need to follow executing the specific dance moves properly. If you are a beginner, look for classes that offer the fundamentals and proper technique in dancing. A lot of dance moves require turnout, it is a form of dance wherein the knees and toes are pointed out to the other side of the body. This type of dance move should not be forced and should be executed naturally.

Injury

If you get to experience dancing, you will be addicted to it. If you have the dance bug, get used to the muscle sores and pulls that you will feel occasionally. Be mindful of the RICE acronym: Rest, ice, compression and elevation. This method will help in the process of quick healing. Remember to take pain relievers like Ibuprofen that can help reduce the pain and eliminate inflammation. Seek medical attention if these medications don't work or if the symptoms still persist. Always remember that if you are exhausted, do not dance for it may cause injuries.

Children

For children that are taking dance classes, remember to hire a reliable and professional dance instructor. A child's bones are still developing and should have the proper training to avoid developing injuries.

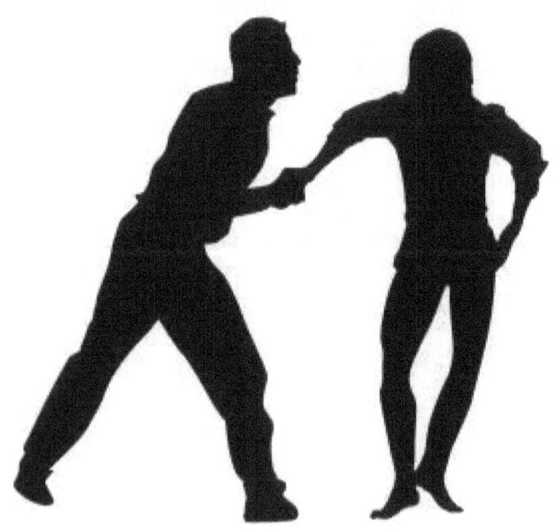

Chapter 5:
The Secrets Behind the Kind of Movements during Dancing and Weight Loss

Synopsis

Dance based workouts have been gaining popularity for a few consistent years now. The reason why a lot of people are getting into it is because it's a lot more fun compared to the high intensity workout you do with the machines you use at the gym. Dancing is very diverse. There are a lot of different types of dances that one can choose from to fit their style and taste.

Other than being a fun and entertaining workout, dancing is proven to be very effective when it comes to weight loss. As a matter of fact, an hour of dancing will allow you to lose as much as 400 calories. This is the same calories you lose if you swim or cycle.

The Secrets

When choosing the right dance workout, one must consider what they want to work on in their bodies. Some dance moves specialize in targeting a certain body part. Some dances will get you to lose weight and others will help on toning muscles.

These dances can be done everywhere! Most people actually go for some facility that holds workshops like a gym, or weekly social dances. Most social dances are held in large restaurants or bars where people can dance with partners. Other people prefer to do it at home where they don't risk getting embarrassed.

If you'd like to know the best dance movements that will burn the calories fast, here are some examples:

Belly dancing - this will target your belly fat, and we know you want to lose the stubborn muffin top. Dancing this regularly will help tone your abdominal muscles and you'll be able to show your flat and sexier belly in no time!

Ballet dancing - Want to tone your muscles but not look bulky? Then this is the dance for you. Not only will you improve your flexibility and have a graceful looking lean body, but you will also have an excuse to wear a tutu!

__Hip hop__ - Have you seen the movie Step Up? If you haven't, it's a must see because it will make you want to start dancing! Imagine having the body of the dancers in that movie. That's motivation enough! Hip hop is a fast paced dance and hits almost all parts of the body. It's both cardio and strengthening.

__Zumba__ - This is a sexy aerobic workout dance making use of music from Latin America. And we all know Latin American dances like salsa, mambo, tango and flamenco are sensual dances. It's also high in intensity; so this cardio will help you lose calories really quick.

__Hoop Dancing__ - This interesting dance uses a hula hoop. Yes, that hula hoop toy you played with as a child is the main star of this dance! There are so many tricks you can learn doing the hoop dance and if you assume that it is only good for your abdominal muscles, then that's where you're wrong. You can use your hoop to target your arms, hips, legs and even knees!

Chapter 6:
Types of Dances Associated with Fat Loss

Synopsis

Dancing is one of the best ways to lose weight. Almost everyone enjoys dancing; those that don't might think of themselves a terrible dancer; therefore lacking the confidence to do it. But dancing can be done anywhere, including the comforts of your own home.

With your favorite music on blast, dancing for a good hour with high intensity can easily burn at least 600 calories; imagine how much weight you can lose if you do it 3-4 times a week. It is a fun and fantastic way to raise your heart rate.

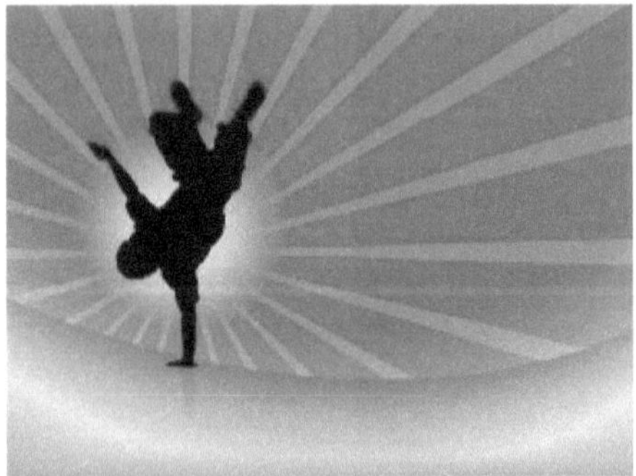

Types

There's no exercise materials involved and there's also no need to lift weights; but you get all the benefits such as strength, toning, flexibility and of course a sexier looking body! There are also different dances to choose from. Some dance styles are harder than others but if you're set on using dancing as your cardio workout, then you can try some or all of them until you find something you enjoy the most.

Belly Dancing

Known to be a very sensual dance, every hip movement targets the strengthening of the core muscles. It also works on improving the body's posture and can prevent any lower back problems. Arms and shoulders are also toned when doing the rippling motions. **An hour of belly dancing will burn 300 calories.**

Zumba

This dance is a total body workout using salsa and merengue music. Like other dance workouts, zumba is a fun way to do your cardio. One of the good things about Zumba is that it's not very repetitive. It has a go with the beat of the music kind of vibe which allows people to feel freer and less routine-like.

Hip Hop

This kind of dance is a form of aerobics but with faster movements. It is also high impact and can help you burn 350 calories per hour. Though it doesn't help too much when it comes to toning muscles, lifting weights might still be necessary if you want to add strength to your training, it's still a good form of exercise.

Hoop Dancing

This is probably the only dance exercise that you'd have to do with a tool which is a hula hoop. It's a unique way to work on your core muscles. For faster weight loss, a heavier hoop should be used but if you want a full dance where you can move faster, a light weight hula hoop should be used. It's not just going to help tone your abdominal muscles though. Hooping in your arms, shoulders, neck and legs are also done and can be learned in class.

There are more types of dance workouts to choose from. What you need to keep in mind though, for better weight loss results is that a balanced diet is always needed. Though these dances are great cardio, eating unhealthy food will lessen the chances for you to shed those extra pounds. Drinking a lot of water and limiting and eating more fruits and vegetables is the best way to go.

Chapter 7:
The Benefits of Fat Loss to Health

Synopsis

Many people, like you and me, live their life stressed and pressured by family, friends, work and even the world itself. All people think of nowadays are the work that needs to be done and their deadlines. Too much stress can lead to poor health. Oftentimes, people tend to forget about their health and neglect the importance of exercise. There are a lot exercises that you can do, and one of the great exercises that will help you stay healthy and fit is dancing.

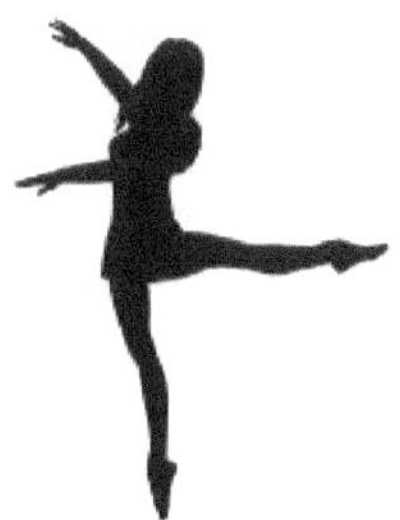

Why Dance

Dancing is considered to be as one of the recommended exercises and activities that will help a person's mind and body become healthier. A person engaged in dancing will reap many benefits, such as enhanced physical agility and mental acuity. Dancing is a fun way to sweat out toxins and fats in your body, while improving an artistic skill set.

It doesn't matter if you are young and old; dancing is enjoyed by everyone of any age. Take some time to observe people that are dancing. You will notice that these people have big smiles on their faces and some are even laughing while dancing. It's because they are having fun while doing it.

There are a lot of advantages that you can get from dancing. The following are the health benefits that you can enjoy from dancing:

- It is good for your lungs and heart
- The muscles on your body will be strengthened
- It will make the bones stronger therefore minimizing the risk of osteoporosis
- It will maximize the body's coordination and spatial awareness
- It increases confidence physically
- It improves mind and nervous system functionality
- Build up energy flow in the body
- Dancing can help reduce weight, will raise social outlook, and will increase self-esteem and overall well-being.

There are many types of dancing. These are jazz, Cuban, salsa, ballet, hip-hop and contemporary. No matter what form of dance you engage yourself, all of them offer equal benefits to the body. You can stick with the dancing genre that best fits your taste, lifestyle and abilities.

Why Lose Fat Now

Losing weight is not just about losing dress sizes; it is about losing fat to improve your BMI or Body Mass Index. It is also about improving your entire life in many significant ways. In fact, studies have proven that losing even just 5% of your body fat can provide the following benefits:

- Lowers high levels of cholesterol in the body
- Improves blood sugar regulation
- Reduces instances of body aches and pains
- Improves mobility
- Improves breathing
- Improves quality of sleep
- Reduces risks of sleep apnea
- Reduces risks of acquiring heart diseases such as angina
- Greatly reduces risks of sudden death caused by stroke or heart diseases

According to research, people who lost just 5% of their body fat have reported great improvements in their quality of life, including emotional health. The study also shows that depression and lethargy has been decreased, providing a more positive outlook to the subjects.

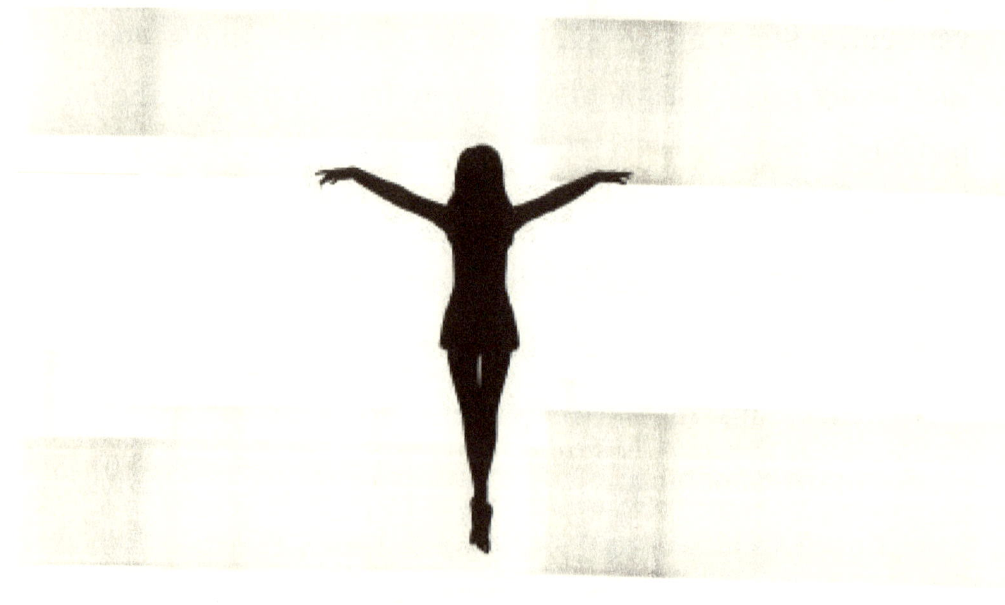

Chapter 8:

How to Avoid Injury

Synopsis

Prevention is still the best cure when it comes to the art – and sport –
of dancing. It may be more fun than other types of fat-burning or
weight-loss activities, but dancing can nevertheless cause you injury
or another type of harm if you are not too careful.

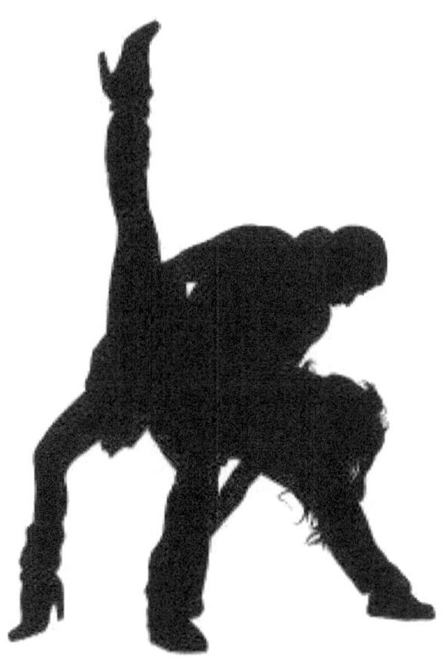

The Most Common Causes of Dancing Injuries

Although the list below is by no means complete, they are by far the most common factors that contribute to dance injuries. Knowing what they are and how they can lead to unfortunate accidents is definitely a good step to take for protecting yourself when dancing.

Type of Dance

Factors such as routines or step variations, the rhythm or tempo being used, and the possible use of additional props and equipment can definitely increase a dancer's risk of being injured. The waltz, for instance, because of its somewhat slow tempo and simple routine, is less "injury-prone" than, say, pole dancing or breakdancing.

Frequency

Simply put, the more times you dance, the higher the risk there is for injuring yourself. The duration of your dancing period also matters.

Attire, Equipment, and Environment

In some countries, their traditional dances require dancers to hold candles in their hands and even balance one on their heads. Obviously, such requirements will make a dancer more prone to injury than usual. As for the environment, consider where you are dancing. Are the floors made of wood or cement? Does the floor have an even surface at least?

Last but not the least, are you dressed suitably for dancing? The right clothes and footwear to use will depend as well on the type of dance you are interested in. Ballet shoes are for ballet while rubber shoes are for hip hop and other similar styles of dancing.

Physical Condition

Dancing can be grueling so it's important that you are reasonably fit and healthy before giving dancing – especially its more advanced forms and complex genres – a try. You should also take care of yourself, increasing your intake of healthy foods and sleeping a regular number of hours each night. Doing so will give you more energy when dancing. Lastly, your medical history will also obviously have an impact on how high the risk for injury is for you.

More Dos and Don'ts for Avoiding Dancing Injuries

- Do consult your doctor before trying out dancing --- especially if are not in tip top condition at present or in the past.

- Do not wear clothing that restricts your movement. Do not "break" your shoes at class.

- Do drink lots of fluids and eat well to keep your energy levels up.

- Do not continue dancing if you experience the most minimal sense of pain.

- Do pay attention to your body limits.

- Do not forget to perform a warm-up before exercising.

- Do read or listen to instructions very carefully to prevent you from making any misstep.

Do not dance without your parents' approval if you are not yet of legal age.

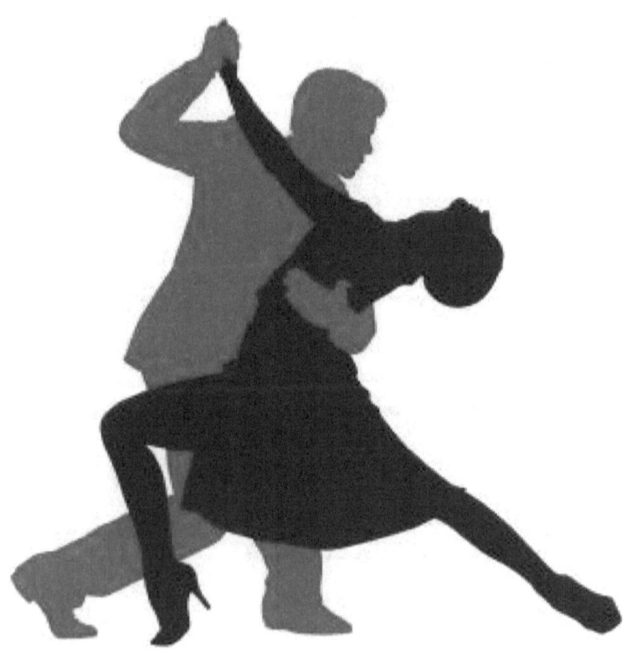

Chapter 9:
The Benefits of Fat Loss to Optimal Health

Synopsis

You may have been advised, at one point or another, to perform aerobic exercise mainly for health and weight management. This type of exercise is important to strengthen your lungs as you increase the oxygen uptake in your body. This will be very beneficial as your cells need continuous supply of oxygen in order to function well.

An aerobic exercise is performed by doing an activity that will allow you to breathe in fresh oxygen and exhale carbon dioxide – a substance that is a by-product from energy usage. With this, you need to do series of light activities like walking, running, jogging, bicycling and many others.

It is also advised to do an aerobe exercise for 30 minutes or so, depending on how your body copes up. Then you can increase gradually as you have adjusted to it. The allowed time is just enough to target all the working muscle groups in your body while providing fresh oxygen to improve your circulatory system. With that, the target heart rate should be increased by approximately 8% so that your heart can efficiently pump up all the nutrients (including the oxygen) throughout your body. This is good to promote lean body mass and sweat the extra calories out.

The Heart Rate Factor

Oftentimes, you will reach an activity level wherein you increase the intensity of your exercise at its peak then slow it down gradually to catch your breath. This is called the aerobic curve and has to be avoided as much as you can. This is because you need to stay at a certain level of heart rate (as mentioned to be an increase of 8%) in order to successfully breathe in the needed oxygen that your body needs during the exercise.

Basically, it is good to maintain a heart rate while doing a light exercise rather than performing it intensely then slowing down after. If you are just starting to do an aerobic activity, it is good to start at a slow pace then increase duration and intensity as you cope up so that you can better avoid an aerobic curve.

Difference from Anaerobic

Anaerobic exercise, on the other hand, is performed at a shorter time but with great intensity. With this, the body makes use of more calories but with lesser oxygen uptake. This type of exercise develops more muscles as it is based on endurance and strength.

This can be performed by sprinting, weight lifting, football, skiing and other intense sports. It also targets the muscles groups and is utilizing more blood and oxygen as compared to aerobic. In short, aerobic exercise supplies more oxygen but anaerobic exercise utilizes oxygen more.

Both aerobic and anaerobic are important to maintain a healthy weight but is dependent on your fitness goal. If you want to lose unwanted pounds and improve your health, then investing more on aerobic exercise is suitable for you. For those who are now well-adapted to exercise at a certain level, it may be time for you to improve your lean body mass and sexy figure with anaerobic exercise.

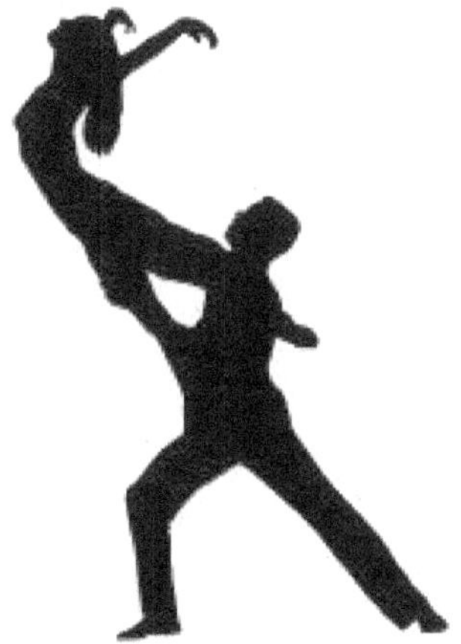

Wrapping Up
Good Lessons to Be Learned From Fat Loss: A Case Study

We all learn from each other. One thing that can keep us going from any challenges is by looking up to someone that was able to achieve something that is similar to our goal. This is particularly true when we are into weight loss. So here is an inspiring story from a case study that will definitely refresh your motivations.

Her name is Angi, a 43 year-old lady who juggles her time as a student and a full time worker. She has a weight of 188.1 pounds or 85.5 kilograms and a total body fat of 41.2%.

This case gave Lee Busby, a fitness instructor who wants to attain a level-3 training qualification, a chance to work on her study. With the help of a nutritionist, Christine Davis, Angi's journey has been a source of inspiration not only from fellow overweight people but to healthcare professionals as well.

Upon initial assessment, Busby determined the sleeping problems of Angi along with physical injuries in the hips and knees. It was also found out that her current program does not really suit her well so it is not effective to give her significant weight loss. This has been followed-up with series of consultations from Davis who gave her a diet plan which Angi can gradually see results in about 8 weeks.

Davis made a new one for her since she followed yet another diet plan that is not really effective. With all these ineffective interventions, Angi became lethargic which led her to have sleeping problems.

Angi's Blog

At the start of her blog, she was glad to have a 12-week program from Busby from a contest that she won, and will meet the fitness team at 12:00 on January 7, 2013. After a tedious assessment and tests, she was given a weekly goal of losing 2 pounds. This can be achieved with daily physical activity and healthy diet. She has to do 6 days of yoga with a diet that is restricted in processed food with lots of water to drink. At this stage, she was explained to have fat loss rather than immediate weight loss.

Her goal is also be able to fit into a tiny bikini as she always admires women who join bikini competition, flaunting their shapes with matching heels. Above all, she still wants to be pregnant despite her age. With that, she promises to endure 12 weeks of strength training and 5-kilometer running to achieve her healthy weight in 6 months. Now, with all the struggles and time juggling, she is now on her way to achieving a healthy weight. Her struggles, ambitions and daily experiences are all in the blog of Berkshire fitness.

Her case is the one that is followed by many health buffs as they see how determined she is to lose weight and get a life she has always dreamed of. With that in mind, it is good to remember that weight loss is never easy. However, the support of credible health professionals and overcoming struggles will eventually lead you to a healthy and happier version of you.

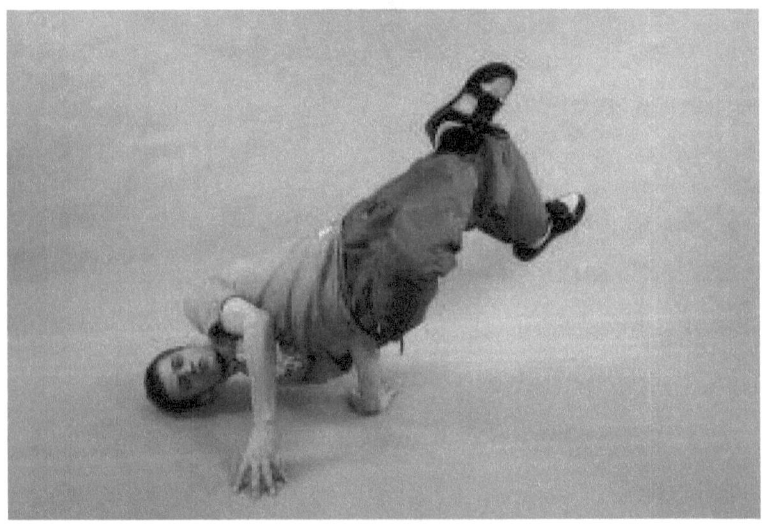